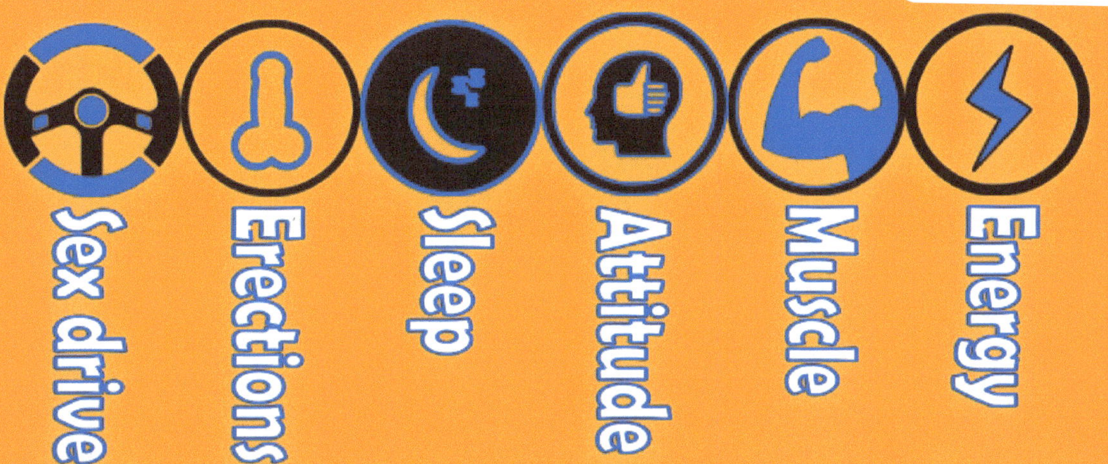

If you are like me you are probably wondering:
-What are my real options?
-Will TRT help me?
-Are Men using this stuff (TRT) or not?
-Is it safe?
-What happens when you take it?

I decided to examine and track my experience with TRT when I could not find real life reviews or evaluations of TRT.

S-E-S-A-M-E

Sesame: is an acronym I invented for several components that I believe are important in a man's life. After I turned 40 I wrote down things I wanted to improve. I wrote down many ideas and wants for my life, but all of it could be lumped in to these 6 things.

Sex Drive, Erections, Sleep, Attitude, Muscle and Energy

Can you remember your twenties? I sure can, and when I was in my twenties I could party all night and then work all day with plenty of energy. Now, at 41, if I partied all night I would literally have to sleep all day. Everytime I would write out what I wanted, like, play more with the kids, or make my wife happy in the bedroom. It would come back to one of these 6 things. So Sesame was born as a way for me to apply data analysis to my health and well being.

I went all the way back to my twenties and started thinking about how I felt and what I could do when I was that age. I lumped the years in 7 year blocks and then averaged the results to get the SESAME total for those years. By doing this I had a chart for my twenties, thirties, and now forties. I could actually make a comparison between the years and how I felt. I could also now forecast how I wanted to feel… and so I picked 29. I am 41 and my goal is to feel and live as though I am 29 again. So SESAME became an obsessionas as I have tried to improve my scores. Over 8 weeks I tracked my SESAME and you will see the real results (Good and Bad) of TRT.

****As a **Bonus** you get exclusive access to the videos series I filmed weekly as I went through TRT (over an hour of content and explanations and demonstrations of what this process is like). Your code is inside the book****

My current Q/L score is 40. Where will I be after 8 weeks?
Was I able to get my 29 year old self back? Find out inside.

Contents

The Mona Lisa is falling apart

One of my favorite lines from *Fight Club* is when Tyler Durden says to Edward Norton's character, "Even the Mona Lisa is falling apart." I was 21 when I watched that movie and had no idea how accurate those lines would be 19 years later.

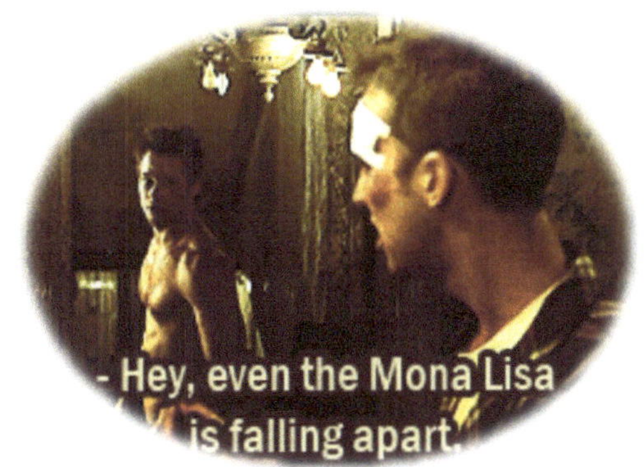

When I was 32 I chipped my right front tooth. I went to the dentist and she said that she could grind the edge off of it but it would be slightly shorter than my other front tooth. As she was grinding away at my tooth I remember thinking, "Even the Mona Lisa is falling apart." It was true. I was getting older and things were bound to happen to me. This event was special to me because it was truly the first time that I was like, "Oh shit, I am going to get older and this might be the best years of my life." Chipped tooth, wrinkles, health issues, might all be on the way, but I was in my thirties and really didn't dwell on it. I had living to do.

As the years went by I stayed in shape because I worked very hard as a wildland firefighter. The daily required PT (Physical

Training) we did kept me in shape unlike many of the other thirtysomethings working in offices. I also met my wife and we had two wonderful children. When my daughter was little I noticed that I was starting to feel a little tired in the evenings and found myself gravitating to the couch instead of playing with her. I was also running a new start up called Rhino Laces and I truly felt like I was burning the candle at both ends.

When my son came along in 2016, I was 38 and struggling in almost every aspect of life that I took for granted in my early thirties. What had happened to me? Was this really how aging was going to be? I resigned myself to working out harder and eating better. I quit gluten and carbs and really became strict on what went in my body. I was convinced that upping my workouts and correcting my diet would return me to my glory. We moved to Hawaii when I was 39 and my son was 6 months old. I also figured the change of pace in Hawaii would improve my mood and sex life. My wife had been saying I had changed. That I was different, more aloof, distant, and cranky. It was true. The harder I tried though the more I seemed to be going backwards. Fast forward to today. I am 41 and have been tracking my health for almost 3 years now. Trying diets and exercise to no avail.

Sex…I have bought devices to help in the bedroom, cock rings, pumps, and sheaths. Some of these things are pretty awesome even if you aren't suffering from erectile dysfunction. You can see my review on these on the website ManRogue.com. However it doesn't matter at all if there isn't any sex drive or desire to begin with. Cialis has been our savior as it allows me to get hard enough to have sex. I have to plan it out though, and there have been many nights I have popped the pill and then gone down stairs and found my wife asleep. I have almost no sex drive. I don't watch porn as I just don't care enough too. The irony is my wife is amazing. In all honesty I find my wife super-hot (She's is 7 years younger and has a perfect body. Seriously I am lucky because she is a 9.8 out of 10) and she loves sex. Like crazy mind breaking sex. We were amazing together for so long and then bit by bit my "Drive" went away. It is one of the most terrible things I have ever gone through.

Muscle…I have been trying creatine again and pre-workout mixes trying to get in better shape, but I all I have managed to do is injure my shoulder, loose about 5 pounds of fat, and gain no additional weight in muscle. I have been a gym guy since I was in college and I really do enjoy staying in shape. The last 2 years have been hard. I workout like I usually do but I just don't have the extra... I don't have a word for it really, but I can describe it as that extra bit of push/drive that gets one more repetition or an extra 5 pounds. This could be energy related or even physiological. I don't know. I have lost my 4 pack (never had a six pack) and chalked that up to age because I still do crunches and workout like I did when I had a 4 pack. So something happened there that I can't explain. I have some fat around my belt line. Just a bit of pudge which is why I only eat tuna for lunch, avoid gluten and sugar, and I don't exceed 1500 calories a day. My diet had been this way for months and I still have the pudge.

Attitude: My attitude is awful and there is stress between me and my wife. She wants me to be more active on the weekends and after work. She wants me to be more active at night after the kids go to sleep. The pressure of letting her and the kids down only adds to my frustration and attitude problems. Each night I wake up around 5 times or more. Then it takes me 10 to 20 minutes to fall back to sleep. The lack of sleep is killing any energy I might have had in the day. This results in me just slogging through the work day only to get home to frustrated kids and a very sex starved wife. Rinse and repeat for the rest of my life.

> "I can't live like this. I have decided that I will change something. I will find something that gets me back my life. The real life that we all deserve."

S-E-S-A-M-E

Sesame: is an acronym I invented for several components that I believe are important in a man's life. After I turned 40 I wrote down things I wanted to improve. I wrote down many ideas and wants for my life, but all of it could be lumped in to these 6 things.   Sex Drive, Erections, Sleep, Attitude, Muscle and Energy.

Everything I was missing in life, and wanted to improve, revolved around those things. Granted I realize that some are codependent on each other such as sleep and energy. However, it is not always true. Can you remember your twenties? I sure can, and when I was in my twenties I could party all night and then work all day with plenty of energy. Now, at 41, if I partied all night I would literally have to sleep all day.   Every time I would write out what I wanted, like, play more with the kids, or make my wife happy in the bedroom. It would come back to one of these 6 things. So Sesame was born as a way for me to apply data analysis to my health and wellbeing.

I went all the way back to my twenties and started thinking about how I felt and what I could do when I was that age. I lumped the years in 7 year blocks and then averaged the results to get the SESAME total for those years. By doing this I had a chart for my twenties, thirties, and now forties. I could actually make a comparison between the years and how I felt. I could also now forecast how I wanted to feel… and so I picked 29. I am 41 and my goal is to feel and live as though I am 29 again.

Each subject below gets a number rating and then the total score is averaged to get the Quality of Life Score or (Q/L)

S=Sex drive (1 to 10)

1 = Never think about sex during the day and want sex once or twice a month.

10 = Sex is one my mind often every day and I want sex twice a day.

E=Erection (1 to 10)

1 = can't get it up at all.

10 = I can punch it through drywall.

S=Sleep (1 to 10)

1= up all night toss and turn.

10= Close eyes and wake up 7 to 8 hours later.

A=Attitude (1 to 10)

1= no desire, no happiness.

10= Happy, can do and overcome anything.

M=Muscle (1 to 10)

Subjective based off your wants. 3 = How I looked at 41.

10= How I looked at 29

E=Energy (1 to 10)

1= can't leave the couch.

10 = even with very little sleep I can still kickass for 24 hrs.

Q/L = (S+E+S+A+M+E)/60

Quality of life age 26

MY 20'S =
UNSTOPPABLE

-I LITERALLY OPERATED A
0462 STIHL MAGNUM
CHAINSAW ALL DAY FOR
ALMOST 2 YEARS.

-I WAS A USFS HOTSHOT
-I WAS A USFS HELI-RAPPELER

Sex drive	=10
Erections	=10
Sleep	=9
Attitude	=9
Muscle	=9
Energy	=10
Q/L	=95

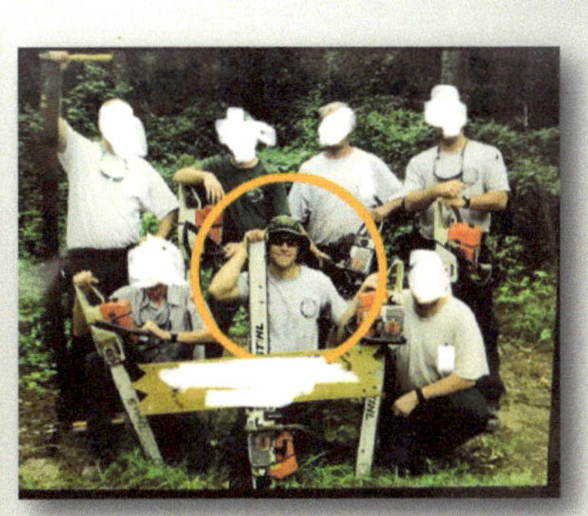

ManRogue

Quality of life age 33

MY 30'S =
STILL A BADASS

-SLOWING DOWN A BIT
-NOT SLEEPING AS WELL
-STILL WANT TO TAKE ON
THE WORLD

Sex drive	=7
Erections	=8
Sleep	=7
Attitude	=8
Muscle	=8
Energy	=7
Q/L	=75

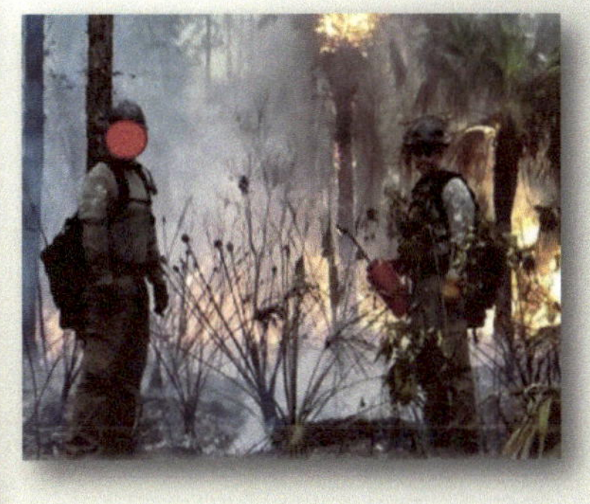

ManRogue

Quality of life age 40

I TURNED 40 =
WTF HAPPENED

-HAVE 2 CHILDREN NOW
-NEVER GET A FULL NIGHTS SLEEP
-NO SEXUAL DESIRE
-LIMP NOODLE
-NOT HAPPY
-HARD TO MAINTAIN MUSCLE

Sex drive =2
Erections =4
Sleep =5
Attitude =4
Muscle =5
Energy =4

Q/L =40

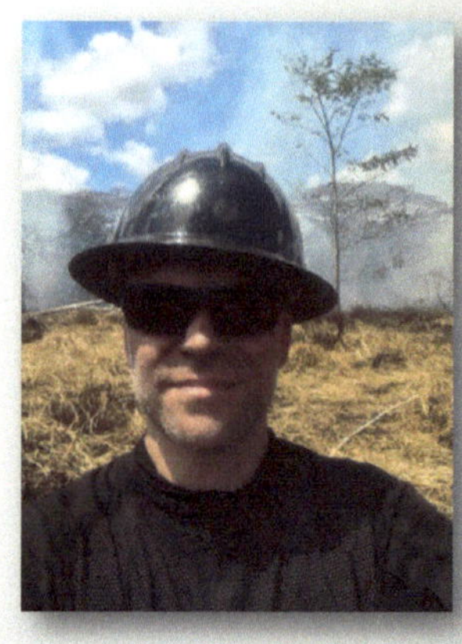

Quality of life age 41

FROM 40 TO 41

-HOLISTIC APPROACHES
-SELF HELP READING
-CIALIS (YEA!!!)
-MEDITATION
-1400 CAL PER DAY DIET

-NEW WORKOUTS

Sex drive =3
Erections =7 (Cialis)
Sleep =4
Attitude =5
Muscle =4
Energy =4

Q/L =45

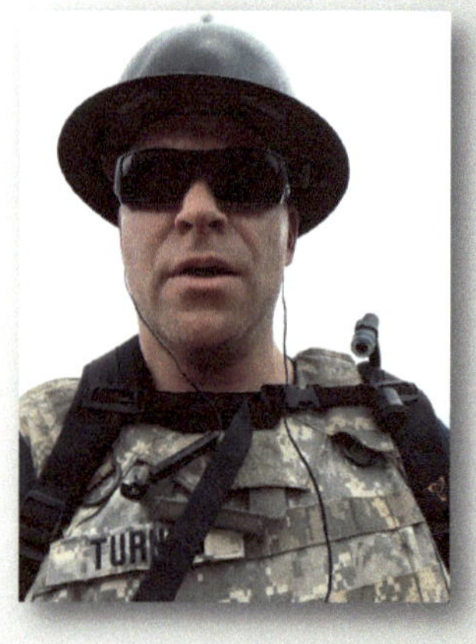

Quality of life age 26	Quality of life age 33	Quality of life age 40	Quality of life age 41
Sex drive =10	Sex drive =7	Sex drive =2	Sex drive =3
Erections =10	Erections =8	Erections =4	Erections =7 (Cialis)
Sleep =9	Sleep =7	Sleep =5	Sleep =4
Attitude =9	Attitude =8	Attitude =4	Attitude =5
Muscle =9	Muscle =8	Muscle =5	Muscle =4
Energy =10	Energy =7	Energy =4	Energy =4
Q/L =95	Q/L =75	Q/L =40	Q/L =45

So what happens now? Is this the best life can get?
I'm barely eating, can't gain muscle, have to take a pill to have a good time, and I can't sleep.

ManRogue

I was able to raise my score by 5 points in one year from 40 to 45. My 26 year old self scored a 95. After a year of self-help books, mediation, diets, exercise, and Cialis I have been unable to really change my Quality of Life score. This sucks. This is not where I wanted to be at 41. I thought I would be killing it like I did at 30. I thought that all these guys that get old, fat and lazy were just genetically unlucky or not trying very hard. Here I am though, I'm in good shape, don't eat junk food, exercise, and only take one pill (Cialis). My doctors are always happy with me because my cholesterol is great, my blood pressure is 120 over 70, and my resting heart rate is around 75. I should be proud of my health, but I am not proud of my life. I am stuck in a life trap.

Physically I am fine but mentally I am a mess. I am depressed, my man parts don't work like they should, and I am tired all the time. So my doctor could only offer me anti-depressants and Viagra. Viagra made me sick so I was switched to Cialis. I don't like pills and didn't want to take an anti-depressant so I didn't. This is the trap I got stuck in when I was 39 and 40. This is also the trap doctors fall in to when trying to diagnose a patient that is physically healthy. Here I am a year later and my quality of life has barely changed.

There is a lot of stuff out there that perpetuates this "Trap":

Viagra and Cialis are #1. It gives a false positive in a world of negatives. It lets you feel just good enough. It doesn't fix the underlying issues. Sure you can get it hard but if you are tired and have no sex drive then who cares. I'm just yawning while thrusting away on my poor wife.

Anti-depressants. The end all be all for mood. My best friend took them and hated it. You become dependent on them and the possibility of a normal life without them becomes harder and harder the longer you take them. It falsely makes you feel better and for some people that is enough. I am not downing people who use them and need them. It just wasn't an option for me after watching my friend struggle with it. I want to feel, but I don't want my feelings to be shrouded or influenced by something I ingest.

Stimulants such as pre-workout, coffee, red bull, or whatever. These were my weakness. I love coffee. I was drinking 7 to 9 espresso shots a day. I would usually have 5 before 9am on days when I was really dragging ass. Redbull I would drink in the afternoon just to stay awake. Often when I got home I would have more coffee at dinner. There is a reason Starbucks and Redbull are multi-million dollar companies. We are all just stealing energy from stimulants just to make it through the day and these companies are genius for tapping in to that need.

The Doctor prescribes us pills and we supply our own stimulants, and we all just slide through life barely making it as we age. Just upping the dose until we die.   Sound ridiculous doesn't it, but that is exactly where I was and how the rest of my life was going to go until a heard a radio advertisement for TRT.

Testosterone Replacement Therapy, the guy on the radio said, would give me back my youth along with some side effects such as acne. Bullshit I thought as I turned my jeep in to the parking lot at my office. Roid rage is not for me and I have had enough acne to last a life time when I was 17.

Several weeks went by and I heard that same advertisement and this time I listened for the name of the clinic. When I arrived at the Fire Cache I got out my phone and looked it up. It was a doctor in his 40's talking about the benefits of TRT and that he too was a patient. Bullshit I thought, just another scam. However, curiosity got the best of me and I decided to investigate this TRT further

I spent all day googling TRT reading reviews and scientific articles. I found so many different opinions from risks to wonderful success stories. The problem was many medical studies contradicted each other and many success stories were from Doctors websites who were just promoting TRT.

In 2013, a study encompassing insurance prescription data on more than 10 million men ages 40 and older from 2001 to 2011 was published in JAMA Internal Medicine. Over that decade, androgen replacement therapy use more than tripled.

Then the trend reversed. Testosterone prescriptions for U.S. men ages 30 and older decreased by 48 percent overall from 2013 to 2016, according to findings published July 10, 2018, in JAMA after researchers revisited the database.

So I was confused are Men using this stuff or not. Is it safe? What happens when you take it? I really wanted an honest testimonial from someone. I could not find one. Many Doctors and businesses out there touting the success of TRT, but no one like me. No regular guy that could provide answers.

I love data. My job requires that I analyze fire weather, fire history, trends, and occurrence data to predict wildfires and forecast fire danger. So I figured I would try to apply this skill to TRT. I will be the guinea pig and tell the world.

This was a perfect opportunity to test my (SESAME) for Q/L (Quality of Life).

My desired outcome is still 29 yr. old self (Q/L of 85%). I will run TRT through SESAME and see what the results are and if TRT is a possible solution for me and perhaps other men like me.

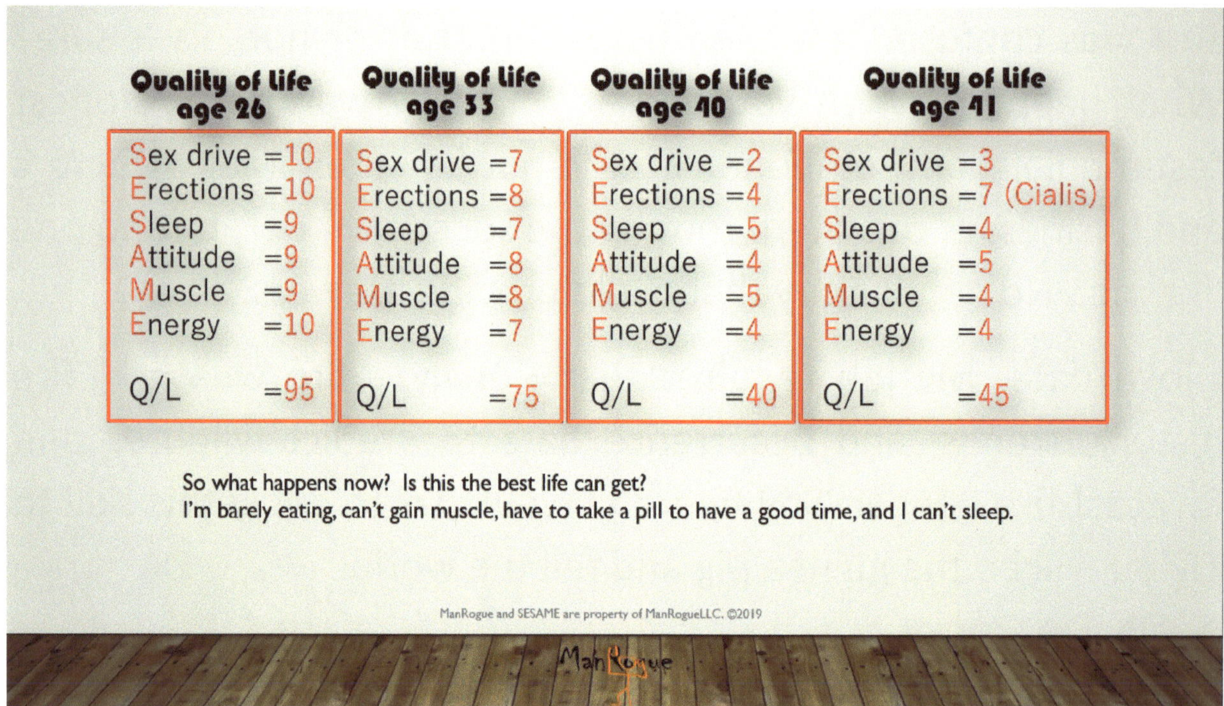

I used
(26yr old Q/L of 95)
+
(30yr old Q/L of 75)
To get an average of 84 for my desired outcome of a 29yr old Q/L.

05/29/2019

I called the clinic that I had heard about on the radio. I was informed by the receptionist that they were booked for weeks. So I said never mind and hung up. I decided it was silly and went back to thinking about other options. I had been feeling a little better and running a little further so maybe I was on to something with my diet and exercise regime.

06/20/2019

I have never been so sore after a workout. I was literally sore for 4 days and to top it off I reinjured my shoulder and my right forearm. Both injuries I have been dealing with for several years. I was angry and mad when I called the Clinic for TRT. The receptionist said they had a cancelation and could see me on the 16th of July. I said I would be there.

As the next several weeks went by I started getting cold feet. Did I really want to do this? What would my wife think? What would my friends and colleagues think?   So one day at work I brought the topic up and almost every single firefighter I work with said they would never do it. That they were fine and didn't need to "take a short cut" or become a roid dude to stay in shape. None of us would ever dare say we had any issues in the bedroom. I agreed with them, but I knew that what I was going through wouldn't go away and I also believed that several of them are in the same boat as me, but they wouldn't admit it. Guys just don't talk about this shit, especially firefighters.

07/16/2019

The day arrived and I made the drive to the clinic. Anticipating super muscular guys and girls would fill the office and gallantly stare at me as I shuffled in. I was pleasantly surprised when I opened the door and saw several older men and a couple young women probably in their 30's. No one took much notice of me as I checked in and waited.

I was taken to a room where a nurse took my pulse and blood pressure and just like always I was a picture of health. She closed the door and shortly after she left the doctor opened the door and introduced himself. He explained that men don't have the amount of testosterone in their 40's, 50's and 60's as they did in their 30's. I said that seems obvious, but what I didn't realize is that we marginalize the loss of testosterone over time, and we can't really see how much we change because it happens over years and not days. I was expecting to get pills or injections and then be sent on my way, but he said they needed 2 separate blood tests and then I would need to come back and have another evaluation to see if I was a candidate for TRT. I told him that my doctor had tested for testosterone back in 2017 and my score was around 600. He said that was mid-range but we still need to do the blood tests again.   So to say I was a little let down when I left his office was an understatement. I was ready to get this going and now I was leaving with a pamphlet on TRT and a script for 2 blood samples.

07/24/2019

I returned to the clinic to find out my results of the blood tests and to see if my liver function was good enough to support TRT. As I walked in the lobby it was a familiar mix of people just like before except for one super big muscular "Rock" looking dude and I thought to myself, "I knew it." They give me my results and my Testosterone levels averaged to 450. 300 or below makes you eligible for insurance to cover TRT because it is considered a serious health issue. I was low and probably within another year would have been below 300. The doctor asked me if I wanted to wait a year. I thought a moment and then asked, "How much is it going to cost without insurance?" He said, "Fifty eight fifty." I said, "five thousand, eight hundred and fifty." He laughed and said, "No its $58.50 for 4 injections… a months' worth". I said, "Sign me up!"

A few minutes later a nurse came in and helped me inject myself in the thigh with testosterone and my journey began just like that.

I am very aware of the placebo effect and that our minds are powerful, but I swear as I drove back home that day the sky seemed bluer, the Hawaiian scenery seemed clearer, and I felt a tinge of happiness and confidence.

You can read all about testosterone and bodybuilding. Those guys are taking huge amounts of testosterone. I am not taking that kind of dose at all. This I had to make clear to my suspicious wife when I got home. My doctor's goal is to get my testosterone back near 900 to 1000. About where most of us are in our late 20's and early 30's. This lines up perfectly with my SESAME 29 year old life I want to live. It will take almost 8 weeks before my Testosterone will average out at those levels so for the next 8 weeks I decided that I will be recording videos and writing about my experiences. I want to be able to explain and show other men like me just what TRT is, and what it may or may not do for you. The good, the bad, and the ugly. I will be as objective as possible because I am looking for truthful answers for ME. It does me, nor my future me, any good to be anything other than absolutely truthful.

Through the whole process I will explain what I feel, and better yet, what SESAME is going on in me. I will log physical changes as well including weight gain or loss. Muscle gain based off the weights I lift and basic measurements of my arms, chest and thighs. I will continue to eat and workout exactly as I did from 40 to 41 so we can truly see if this is working. With one exception. I now drink Vodka with a splash of club soda, and pineapple juice instead of IPA's…So a few less calories.

Starting numbers for SESAME

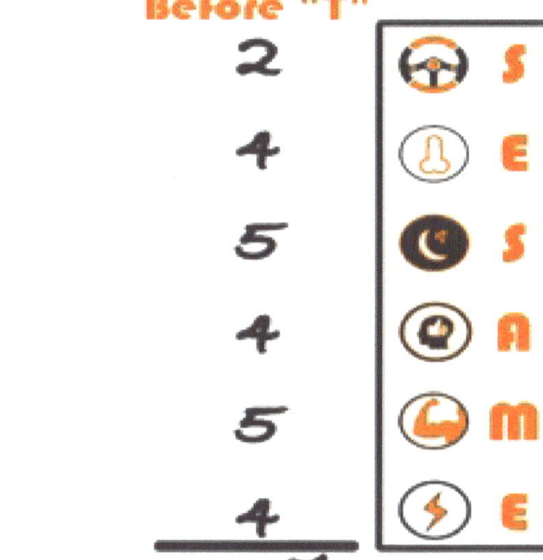

Biceps= 13.5	
Quads= 21.5	
Chest= 40	

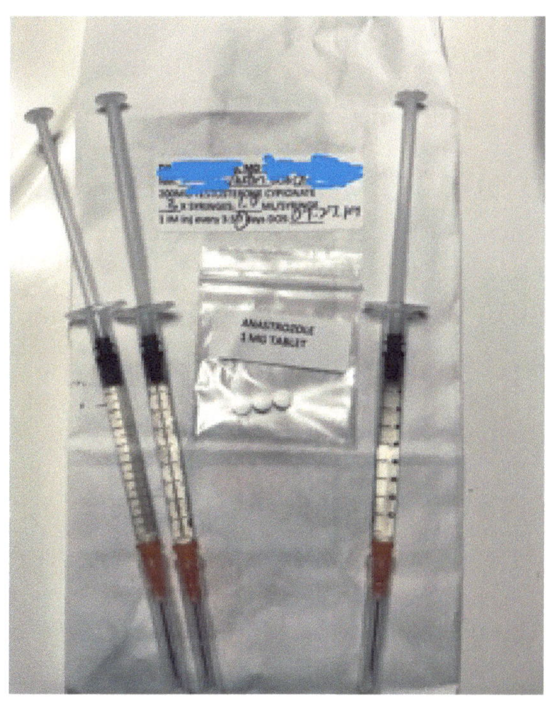

TRT 8 Week Experiment

Week 1 was interesting. I want to feel different but other than some cool dreams I haven't noticed really any changes.

Sex drive: Still shitty as before. Hardly ever feel aroused or want sex

Erections: This needs to improve. Without Cialis it's barely hard enough to penetrate her.

Seep: The first thing I noticed that got a little better. I am waking up only one time a night now versus like 5 so that's good.

Attitude: This too had been different. A little bit more motivated. I put it up there at the 6 to 7 range where I haven't been that way in probably three or four years. Along with the attitude I am a little bit more motivated, a little bit clearer. I played with my kids last night and I haven't done that in a while, and the day before I took them out to the park. Before when I got home from work I just kind of wanted to eat and chill.

Muscle: Too soon to tell. Still sore after workouts and look the same as before.

Energy: I don't expect this to really change but we will see. I have never found anything that states TRT will give you energy. Still about the same.

Negatives:

I've had a little bit of a headache in the mornings and when I get up.   It feels like a hangover. I've read that when you start this you should be hydrating a little more than usual and I haven't been doing that.

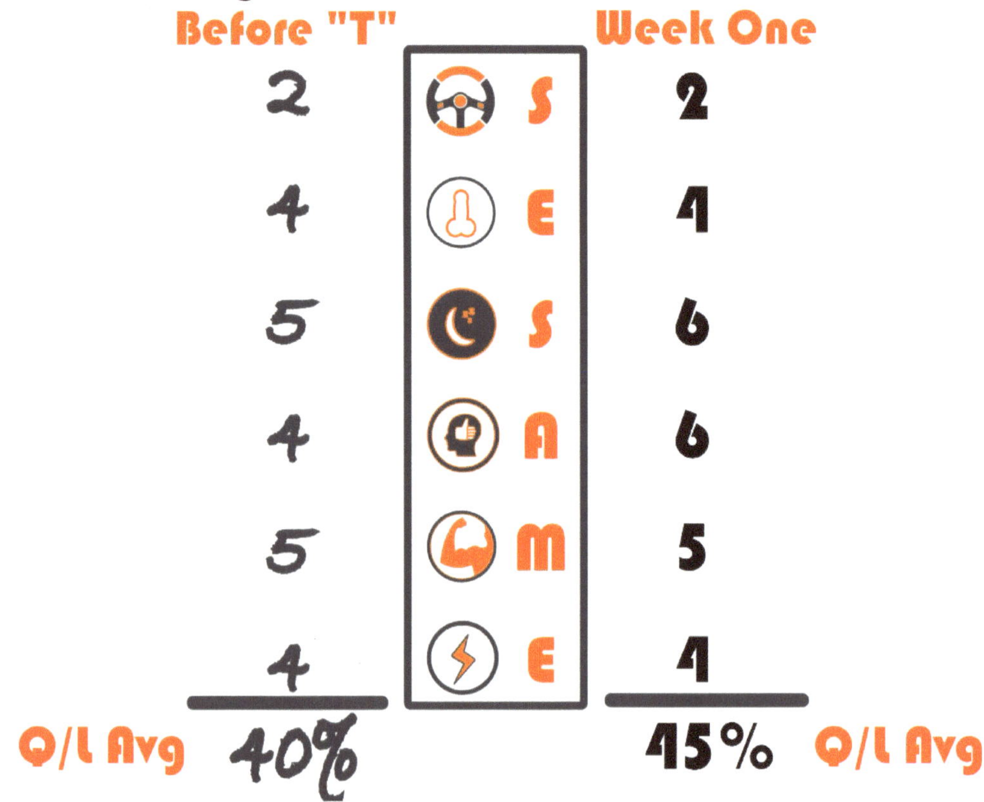

Week 2 and 3:

I'm through week 3 and I am starting to see and feel some pretty cool changes.

Sex Drive: My Sex Drive has increased. I have wanted sex about 3 to 4 times a week. And I would estimate that my Sex Drive is about a 5 to 6 right now.

Erections: My dick is doing better. I woke the other night at 2am. and I wanted to have sex with my wife.   We were spooning so I woke her up. I was decently hard (Without Cialis) I would say it was a 5 to 6 on the erection scale. After about 20 minutes I became very soft and could no longer stay in her. She was happy that she got to have her Big "O" twice, but she was not excited that I went limp. This is the psychological shit that she has been dealing with and she usually feels as though there is something wrong with her.   There must be something wrong with her otherwise I would always be hard and always be able to cum. It really sucked trying to go back to sleep that night. I wanted to please her but I also wanted her to see that this TRT was working, and thus proving that our sex difficulties were all my fault these past 2 years and not hers. However, we only proved that I was able to perform semi successfully with a semi hard dick for about 20 minutes.   Usually we would use cock rings and other items to keep me going but we ended our night of fun and just accepted it for what it was. Not perfect, but a little better.

Sleep: Sleep has been good.   I was awaking up with an occasional boner and I was starting to have more energy but that might be due to good sleep. Fortunately with my career I work 24 hours on including overnight, and there are many nights I hardly sleep so I will be able to judge if it is TRT that is increasing my energy, or if my increased energy is actually from just improved sleep. All in all I would say sleep is at a 7 or 8.

Attitude: has been much better I and would dare say near an 8. I am happier and more engaged in life, not just work but also family life.

Muscle: It's improving. My wife said I lost the baby. Which was insulting but I know what she means. The little pudge is starting to recede from around my waist. She said my pecs are becoming more defines again and my arms look better. I haven't been sore after workouts. So I plan to up my workouts to 1.5 hours instead of 1 and see what happens. Muscle is a 6.

Energy: as mentioned before I need some more time to see if TRT is the cause of this energy increase or just improved sleep.

Negatives: Occasionally I have a morning headache. I am trying to be aware of how much water I drink throughout the day and I am drinking as much as I always have the headache is a side effect.

Before "T"
Week Three
2   S   5.5
4   E   5.5
5   S   7.5
4   A   8
5   M   6
4   E   4
Q/L Avg   40%   61%   Q/L Avg

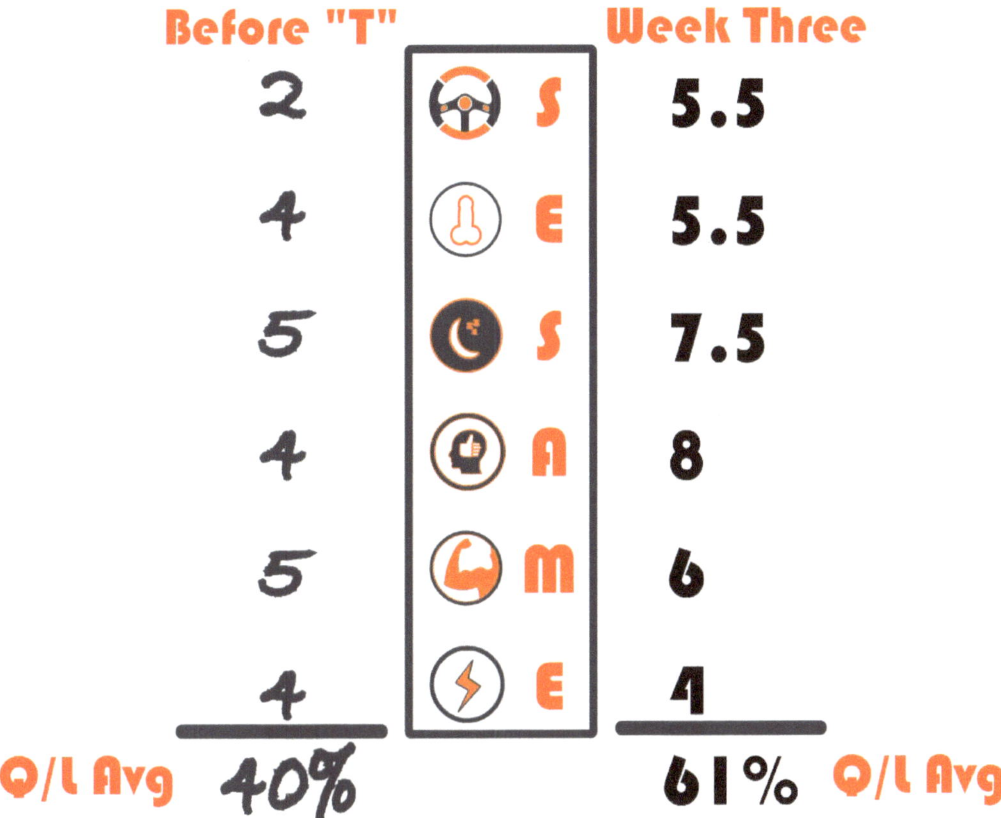

From week 4 to the end of week 5 it has been awesome. I have really noticed some differences that are making me think this whole TRT thing might be worth it.

Sex Drive: My Sex Drive has greatly increased. I have wanted sex about 1 to 2 times a day. And I would estimate that my Sex Drive is about a 7 to 8 right now.

Erections: My dick is doing fantastic. My erections are lasting as long as I need them to. My wife even said my dick felt longer and thicker which gave me a huge confidence boost but also makes sense as she has only been getting a semi hard cock for almost 3 years.   Now it's fully functional and is getting exceptionally hard.   Still not my 29 year old hard on, but damn close. So right now my boners are at an 8

Sleep: Sleep has been pretty good. I mentioned before that I work some crazy shifts and I got 2 of such shifts over the last 2 weeks. I slept about 4 hours but was constantly interrupted sleep either by the radio going off or checking the fire we were on. The next day I was feeling the lack of sleep for sure. I'll talk more about this in the energy section. Regular night's sleep are very good and are at an 8.

Attitude: I am taking more initiative and also seem generally more positive. My attitude is still at an 8 but so much better than where I started.

Muscle: I have been going to gym 3 times a week and have seen decent gains in all the lifts that I do. I have been extending my workouts to 1:15 and 1:30. I do legs twice a week and chest once a week because I read that building your legs and quads also help with natural testosterone production. Muscle is a 7.

Energy: So it appears that TRT does help with my overall energy. As mentioned above in the sleep sections. I didn't sleep much for two nights and the next day I could feel that I was mentally fatigued but my body was good to go. I was able to keep going without coffee or stimulants and I generally had about 85% of the energy I usually would after a great night's sleep.   My general day to day energy levels are at an 8.

Negatives: Started upping my water intake and no more headaches. So make sure you drink more than you need. You should Pee often and Pee clear. If not then drink water. I did get pretty angry at my daughter and yelled at her in the kitchen without too much provocation. My wife said it was extreme and instantly accused me of roid rage. Well shit. I knew the first time I got angry or upset that this would happen. People always assume that roid rage happens to anyone taking testosterone. Although I don't think I am taking anywhere near enough to cause that. I don't know if it has anything to do with TRT or not. I will see if it becomes a pattern.

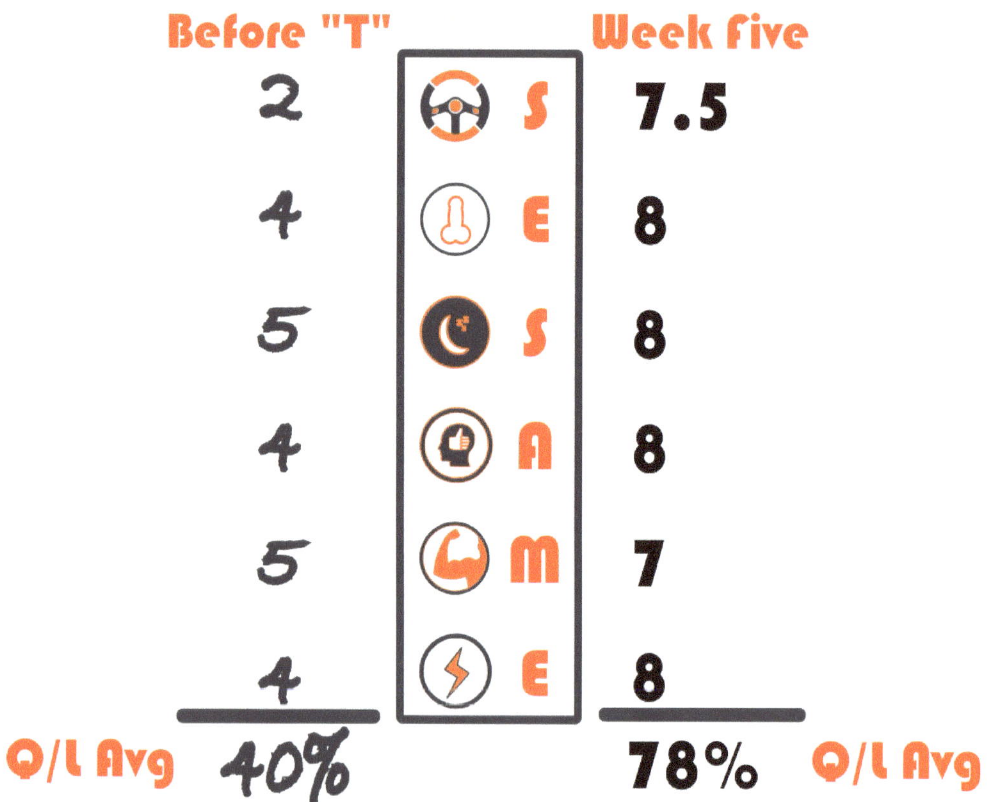
Before "T"
Week Five
2
S
7.5
4
E
8
5
S
8
4
A
8
5
M
7
4
E
8
Q/L Avg
40%
78%
Q/L Avg

From week 6 to the end of week 7 I have come to realize that I should have started TRT 5 years earlier. My whole life and outlook on life has improved

Sex Drive: My Sex Drive is just like I was in my late teens to early twenties. WOW! I have wanted sex about 4 to 5 times a day. And I would estimate that my Sex Drive is about a 9 to 10 right now. Seriously my wife just brushes by me and I smell her perfume and I want to rip her clothes off her body. This has been great but must be exercised with caution. Too much is still too much. I am trying to match her sex drive that is now less than mine. I don't take it personally if she doesn't want to. We have more than enough sex to make me and her happy. That was the goal. I will say that any time she wants to fuck, make love, have sex, or just dry hump that I would be ready to go in an instant. My sex drive is back and always ready.

Erections: This is my favorite as my boners are fantastic now. I would say they are at the 9 level… almost a ten. So I cheated a bit and took 5ml of Cialis the other night and it was a perfect 10.   Hard as ever and it worked and felt amazing for all involved.   My orgasm was even longer and more intense. Fucking sweet.

Sleep: Sleep is still an 8. So much better than week 2 but not perfect sleep where you just don't wake up until the alarm goes off. I have had some incredible and vivid dreams though. This tells me I am entering REM sleep and my mind and body is at rest.

Attitude: My Attitude is now a 9 easily. It could be my massive boners, or the good sleep, or the fact that my wife is happy with me, or that my muscle is returning, or all of this but I am unstoppable right now.

Muscle: I am still going to gym 3 times a week and I am still not getting sore after a workout which means I could workout more often. Yesterday I felt a twinge of pain while doing squats and I stopped. I learned in life regardless of TRT or not that pain in the gym should be listened to. I have nothing to prove. I just want my body in good shape. I am getting there. I am still a 7 but getting better and a little bigger every day.

Energy: Energy is still an 8. I have not noticed any increase or decrease these last 14 days.

Negatives: Still no more headaches. Sensitive to loud noises but I could just be getting old. Have found myself feeling a little more irritable with dumb people and dumb shit. Might be related to TRT.

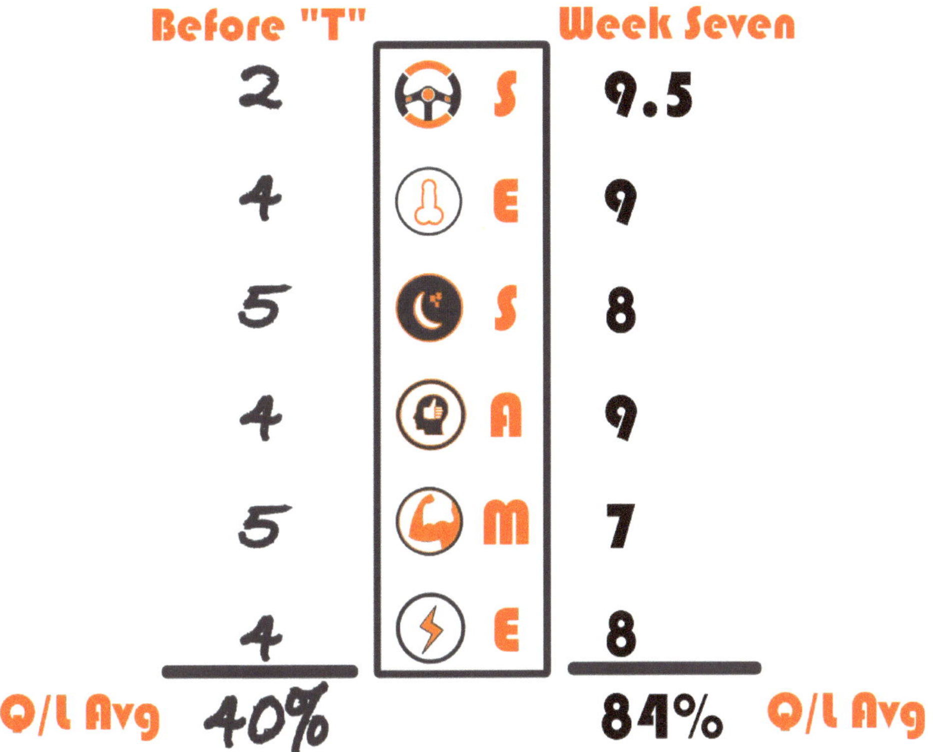

Before "T"
Week Seven
2   S   9.5
4   E   9
5   S   8
4   A   9
5   M   7
4   E   8
Q/L Avg   40%   84%   Q/L Avg

09/21/2019

This is my last week before going to see the Doctor and having my TRT levels analyzed with blood tests. We will find out if my level is ideal, low or high.

Sex Drive: My sex drive is now a 10. I want sex probably too much, but I wouldn't change that for a minute. If you're married talk with your wife. My wife is understanding and I tease her that she got what she asked for. However for my age I think that having sex once a day is phenomenal. I however, want sex 2 to 100 times a day. Literally we could be deep cleaning our bathrooms and I look over at my wife all bent over scrubbing the tub and boom, suddenly all I can think about is her naked spread out on the bathroom floor. In turn this leads to a very obvious erection and then my wife looking at me like I am a sex crazed 19 year old. Although there is something hot about getting it on in the middle of the day on a freshly cleaned bathroom floor or counter. As I write this I am going to need to take a break and see if she wants to clean something.

Erections: 9 without Cialis and a 10 with Cialis. Still a great combo to put together but most days I just go without Cialis. My dick has not been able to be erect and hit my belly while standing up in almost 10 years. Now I am always poking my belly button when I get hard. This is obviously exciting for me but my wife loves the visual representation of my desire for her. It's great.

Sleep: Sleep is still an 8. This may because of having young kids and always listening even when asleep for them. I hear my son get up at night and go potty or my daughter coughing with cold. So I am happy with an 8. Perhaps it will get better but I can't complain.

Attitude: My Attitude is a strong 9. I feel great and want to do more stuff. I am aware that I don't have the blind ignorance I did at 29 so maybe my attitude is based off real life and not bullshit when I was 29 and my attitude was 10.

Muscle: It has started to happen. I am seeing definition and I am lifting more weight without getting sore. I have more energy and can lift longer. I have lost some body fat. I hope to lose more but I am getting there and my wife loves my body again. She says I look like I did when we met. I give Muscle an 8 now.

Energy: Energy is still an 8. I have not noticed any increase or decrease these last 14 days.

Negatives: I want sex too much. I know I can't have it both ways. I would always prefer to want sex too much, rather than not at all. I keep telling my wife I am making up for all the missed opportunities that her and I should have had. I just have to be aware that it is not fair to expect to make it all up in one week. But I would love to try.

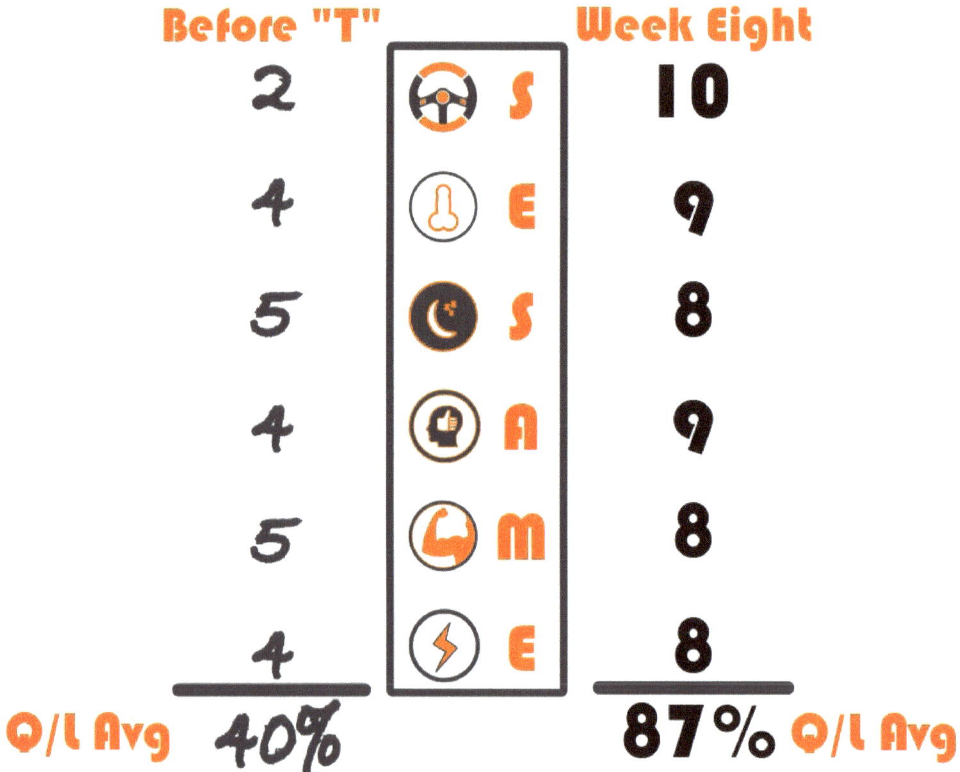

Before "T"
Week Eight
2
4
5
4
5
4
10
9
8
9
8
8
S
E
S
A
M
E
O/L Avg 40%
87% O/L Avg

Culmination

So I know it's easy to read this and listen to my rankings and either think I am full of shit, paid to say these things, or just lucky. I am none of that. I wanted to tell my story honestly and I have. Maybe you think this won't work for you or perhaps you're not as bad as I was. Well that was me from 35 to almost 42 years old. I believed it would all come back. I believed I could get it all back if I just worked harder, or took more supplements or just tried harder in my relationship. Feel free to try, and I hope it works out for you.

In the event that it doesn't work out for you I hope you know there are other options. I swear by TRT now. I am a believer, and I can't believe every male with low testosterone is not doing this. Why live a half life when you can live a full life. Go see the doctor. Make an appointment and see what can be done. This has saved not only my future self but my marriage and relationship with my kids.

I plan to continue TRT and will update once a month as I continue to go through life and living it as fully and completely as possible. This can also be found at ManRogue.com. The doctor told me that the mental improvements tap out at week 7 and 8. That is fine by me as I have greatly improved in this area. He also stated that my physical performance and muscles would continue to improve and reach its peak around the 11th month so I will be keeping track of that progress as well.

Would I recommend TRT. Hell yes. My goal was to be at 84%. I am now at 87% with the potential to go higher. I truly hope this has been helpful for you. I wish I could have found something like this as it would have made my decision to use TRT easier. I may have even started TRT years earlier if I had known this information. I wish you the best and please join us and fell free to share your stories on ManRogue.com.

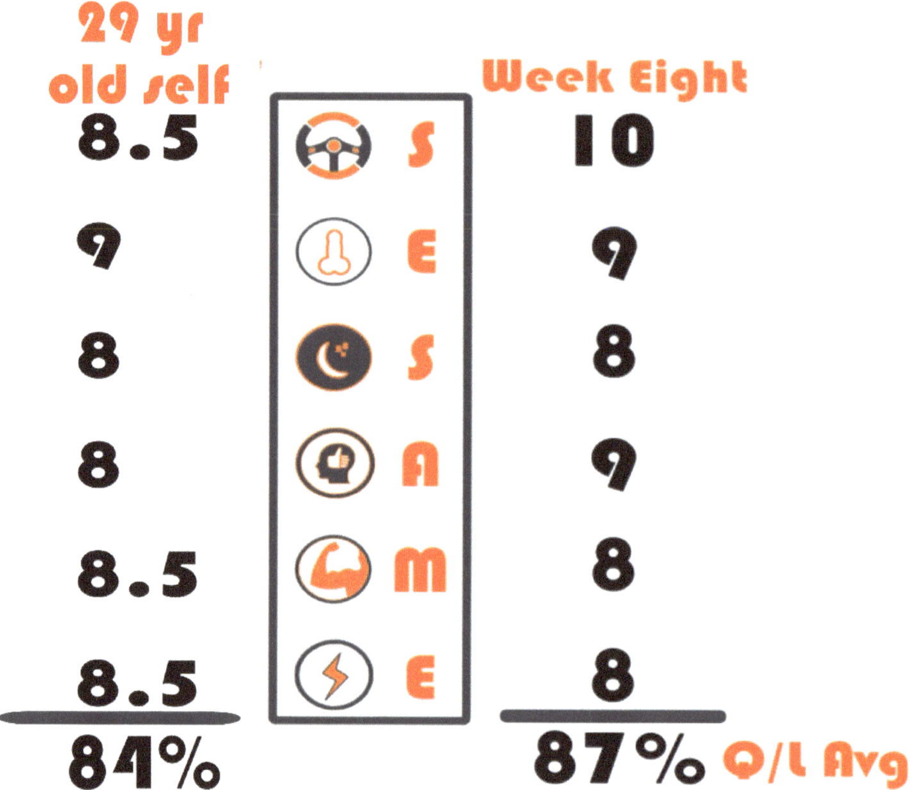

Starting numbers for SESAME	
Biceps= 13.5	
Quads= 21.5	
Chest= 40	

After 8 weeks of TRT	
Biceps= 15.75	
Quads= 22	
Chest= 40.5	

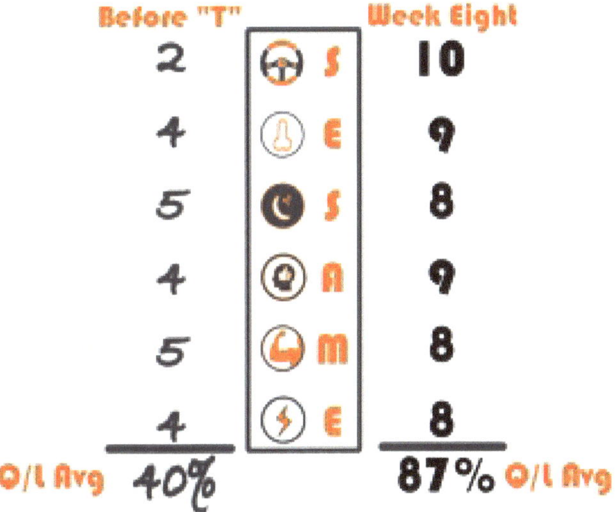

Also please feel free to leave a positive review on

[this book on Amazon](#)

if it helped you make a decision about TRT

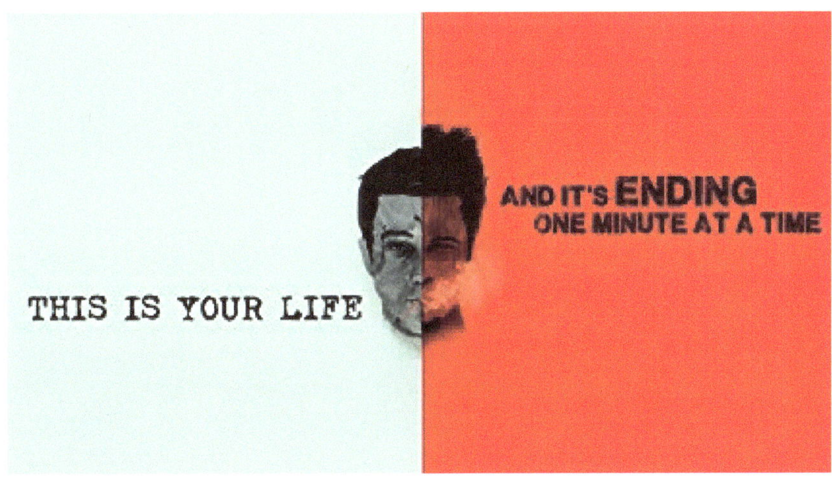

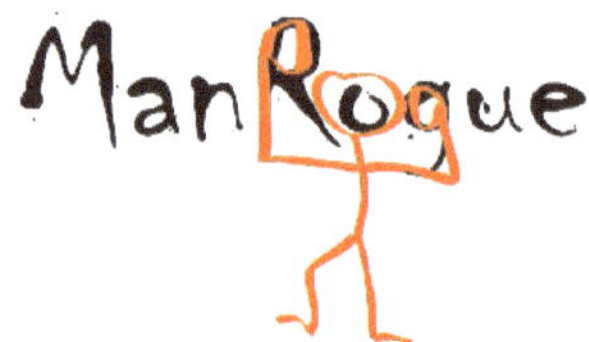

I started Manrogue.com to share my story as an aging male, but it has become so much more than that for men over the age of 37. It is a place to share tips and learn in a pretty cool environment. We are always welcoming new members and new contributors. If you have any tips or lessons for life you can become a contributor and your membership is free.

As a contributor it doesn't matter if it is video content or writing, we help you through the process and create your webpages, videos and ebooks, etc for free. You get 87% of all sales and ads revenue on your topics etc. We brand you and you represent our brand ManRogue.

Email us Manrogue7@gmail.com Subject: Contributor

I look forward to the next 40 years and sharing all the ways we find to keep improving with age.

We owe it ourselves gentlemen.

FOR YOUR EXCLUSIVE ACCESS TO THE VIDEO SERIES PLEASE CLICK HERE:

https://www.manrogue.com/trt-videos   Password: TRTBOOK

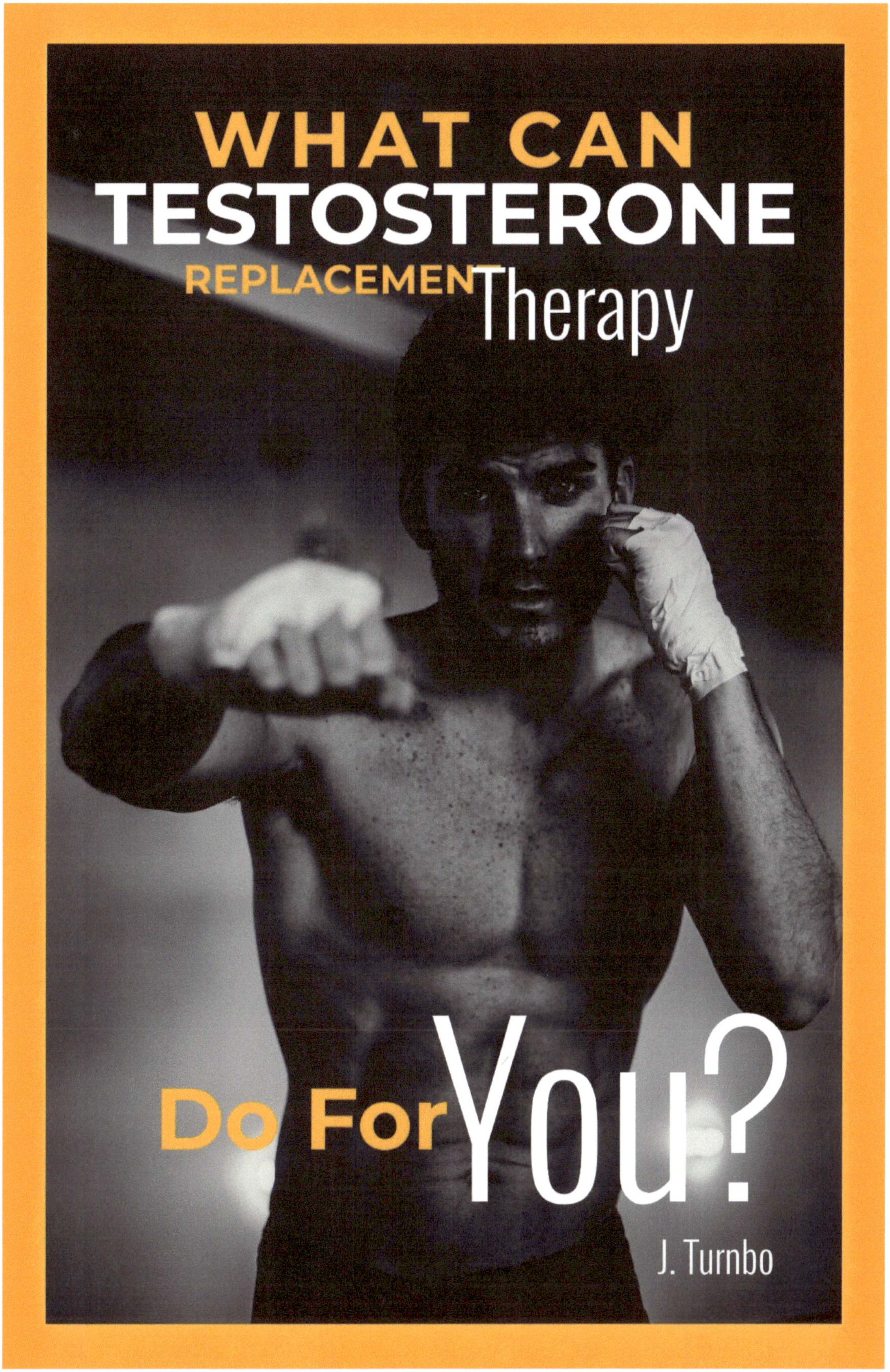

WHAT CAN
TESTOSTERONE
REPLACEMENT Therapy
Do For You?
J. Turnbo